Diabetic Smoothies

35 Delicious Smoothie Recipes to Lower Blood Sugar and Reverse Diabetes

Amanda Hopkins

© **Text Copyright 2020 by Insight Health Communications - All rights reserved.**

This document is geared towards providing exact and reliable information in regards to the topic and issue covered. The publication is sold with the idea that the publisher is not required to render accounting, officially permitted, or otherwise, qualified services. If advice is necessary, legal or professional, a practiced individual in the profession should be ordered.

From a Declaration of Principles which was accepted and approved equally by a Committee of the American Bar Association and a Committee of Publishers and Associations.

In no way is it legal to reproduce, duplicate, or transmit any part of this document in either electronic means or in printed format. Recording of this publication is strictly prohibited and any storage of this document is not allowed unless with written permission from the publisher. All rights reserved.

The information provided herein is stated to be truthful and consistent, in that any liability, in terms of inattention or otherwise, by any usage or abuse of any policies, processes, or directions contained within is the solitary and utter responsibility of the recipient reader. Under no circumstances will any legal responsibility or blame be held against the publisher for any reparation, damages, or monetary loss due to the information herein, either directly or indirectly.

Respective authors own all copyrights not held by the publisher.

The information herein is offered for informational purposes solely, and is universal as so. The presentation of the information is without contract or any type of guarantee assurance.

The trademarks that are used are without any consent, and the publication of the trademark is without permission or backing by the trademark owner. All trademarks and brands within this book are for clarifying purposes only and are owned by the owners themselves, not affiliated with this document.

ISBN: 978-1-64842-044-3

Table of Contents

Introduction Of Diabetic Smoothies 1
    The Diabetic Diet 1
    Diabetes Superfoods 3
    How Smoothies Can Help 3
    Tips to Making Delicious Smoothies 4

Recipes For Diabetic-Friendly Smoothies 6
    1. The Great Green Smoothie 6
    2. Cuke and Kiwi Smoothie 7
    3. Straw-Celery Smoothie 7
    4. Bloody Mary Smoothie 8
    5. Carrot and Ginger Smoothie 9
    6. Thanksgiving Smoothie 9
    7. Cabbage Patch Smoothie 10
    8. Vegetable Soup Smoothie 11
    9. It's All Greek to Me Smoothie 11
    10. Veggie Madness Smoothie 12
    11. Health and Healing Smoothie 13
    12. Eat Your Spinach Smoothie 13
    13. Kale and Cantaloupe Smoothie 14
    14. Pumpkin Patch Smoothie 15
    15. Salsa Smoothie 15
    16. Pizza Smoothie 16
    17. Cucumber-Pear Smoothie 17
    18. Bitter Melon Smoothie 17
    19. Minty Cantaloupe Smoothie 18
    20. Nutty Blackberry Smoothie 19
    21. Greenberry Smoothie 19
    22. Creamsicle Smoothie 20
    23. Greek Grapefruit Smoothie 21

24. Cran-Apple Smoothie 21
25. Peachy Keen Smoothie 22
26. Bluest of Berries Smoothie 23
27. Nutty Pear Smoothie 23
28. Cinnamon Pear and Apple Smoothie......................................24
29. Citrus Smoothie 25
30. Kiwi and Strawberry Smoothie 25
31. Chunky Apricot Smoothie 26
32. Ginger and Turmeric Smoothie 27
33. Orange Juicy Smoothie...27
34. Sensational Spices Smoothie 28
35. Coconut Almond Smoothie 29

Conclusion 30
Check Out My Other Books 31

Introduction Of Diabetic Smoothies

While diabetes is a condition that no one wants to have, it's something that can be proactively managed through your lifestyle and what you eat. There is no reason to think you can't have a full, productive and joyful life just because you have been diagnosed with diabetes. In this introduction of diabetic smoothies, you will learn that smoothies can be a welcome and beneficial part of your diet.

The Diabetic Diet

Diabetics have a higher than normal blood sugar level. The pancreatic hormone, insulin, helps body cells to use glucose for energy. Diabetics either don't produce enough insulin (type 1), or their cells do not respond to insulin like they should (type 2). As a result, the person's blood is flooded with glucose. Glucose in and of itself is not bad, but when its levels in the bloodstream get too high, it damages the kidneys, nervous system, skin, eyes, and cardiovascular system. If you have diabetes, you need to be especially careful of what you eat. There are certain foods that you need to embrace and avoid when you are trying to keep your diabetes under control.

Refined sugar is something to be avoided. This is commonly found in junk food that you already know is bad for you: cakes, cookies, ice cream and doughnuts. Most people don't realize that sugar is added to a lot of other packaged and processed foods. Things that seem innocent and even healthy, such as canned soups, cereals and yogurts can sometimes have unhealthy levels of sugar added to them. Read your labels before you buy something and eat it.

Carbohydrates are also something you should watch when you have diabetes. Since we need carbohydrates for energy, it is not advised that you remove them from your diet totally. Diabetics should aim for 30 to 60 grams of carbohydrates per meal, and 15 to 30 grams for snacks. However, since people respond to carbohydrates differently, the best way to check is to test yourself after each meal.

The carbohydrates you eat should come from high fiber foods and whole grains. Don't eat simple carbs because they will only disrupt your blood sugar and make it harder for you to stay healthy. Chips, pretzels and white bread might all seem okay since you don't associate those foods with sugar. However, your body will metabolize the carbohydrates and turn those ingredients into glucose.

Fruits and vegetables are good dietary staples for people with diabetes. The fiber they have helps slow down the absorption of glucose in the body. They are low in calories, and they will also help you control your appetite. For example, you can satisfy your sweet tooth with a bowl of fresh berries or toss these ingredients into a smoothie.

Fruits and vegetables contain important antioxidants, vitamins, minerals, fiber and other nutrients. They also have a lower glycemic index than a lot of other foods, so you can incorporate them into your diet without disrupting the glucose levels in your body. Fruits and vegetables do contain carbohydrates and sugars, but they are natural ingredients, which makes them safer and healthier. Nearly all doctors, nutritionists and even the American Diabetes Association promote fruits and veggies as valuable parts of the diabetic diet.

Choose the Type of Fats You Eat

Not all fats are created equal, there are good fats and bad fats. This is important to note as diabetics have an increased risk of heart disease and strokes. Watching the type of fats you consume will be part of your diabetes diet.

Trans fat and saturated fat are bad for the heart. Processed meat such as hotdogs have high contents of saturated fat. When buying food in the grocery, the amount of trans fat is specified in the label. Trans fat is present in some processed snacks or junk food, baked goods, margarines - and you should avoid them completely.

The good fats include monounsaturated or polyunsaturated fats. They are found in avocado, olive oils and most nuts.

In addition to vegetables, fruits and good fats, **protein** is an important part of a diabetic diet. So fill up on beans, fish, eggs, chicken and lean beef.

Diabetes Superfoods

Studies have shown that some foods and spices are especially helpful in lowering blood sugar. These diabetes superfoods include celery, bitter melon, pumpkin, tomatoes, spinach, berries, nuts, and cinnamon. These superfoods can help improve the body's sensitivity to insulin, repair damaged cells in the pancreas, and reduce blood sugar levels.

How Smoothies Can Help

The introduction of diabetic smoothies into your diet can provide you with many benefits. First of all, they are delicious. When you're watching what you eat and trying to stay healthy, it's easy to feel deprived. Your mind can trick you into thinking you're hungrier than you are because you're not indulging in the rich desserts or easy snacks that you might have consumed in the past. A smoothie can be a meal, a snack a dessert or something quick that you grab on the go.

You'll feel less deprived, and that will help you control cravings and binges.

Smoothies also provide you with nutrients and vitamins. All of the healthy ingredients that are found in fruits and vegetables are present in smoothie form. You can capture the cancer-fighting antioxidants, the vitamins that improve your immune system and the minerals that make you stronger and keep you healthy.

When you include smoothies in your diet, you're able to control your blood sugar. If you find yourself getting hungry and needing something good to eat, you don't necessarily have to head to the kitchen to cook up a meal. Instead, you can throw just a few fresh or frozen ingredients in a blender, and you'll be able to balance your blood sugar. You'll feel better, stay in control and give your body a boost of exactly what they need. The convenience factor cannot be overstated. It only takes you a few minutes to make a smoothie. If you're trying to keep your entire family on track, you can make four or five smoothies at one time as easily as you can make just one.

Tips to Making Delicious Smoothies

One of the first things you'll need is a blender or a smoothie maker. There are hundreds of different models available in all price ranges. If you don't currently have a blender, invest in a good one. To control and manage your diabetes, you'll want to make a lot of smoothies on a regular basis, which means you need a reliable and easy to use machine.

Next, make sure you use high quality ingredients. If you want a great tasting smoothie, you need to use great tasting foods. You can use fresh fruits and vegetables that are seasonal and abundant. Scout out your local farmer's market to see what's good. If you aren't able to access fresh fruits and vegetables, another option is frozen foods. These are often more affordable, and you can buy things like frozen blueberries and carrots all year long.

Decide what you're looking for in a smoothie texture. Some people like them very smooth and others like to add a lot of ice cubes to provide a chunky, nearly frozen treat. You may need to experiment a little bit to find the texture that really works well for you. It's important to enjoy the process as well as the final result, so don't look at this as a chore. Consider it another tool in your diabetic toolbox.

Hopefully, this introduction of diabetic smoothies will make you excited to try the diabetic-friendly smoothie recipes in this book. These smoothies will help you deliver all the fruits and vegetables that you need, and if you don't love cooking them - this is a great option for you. Smoothies are enjoyed by everyone, and there's no reason for you to miss out on them just because you have diabetes.

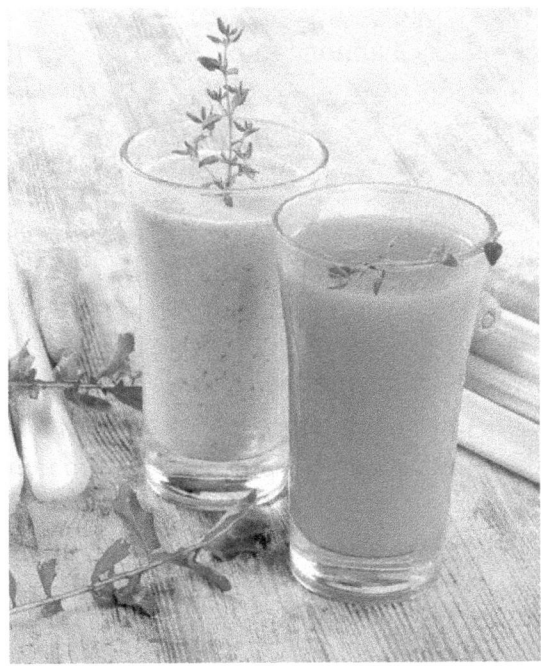

Recipes For Diabetic-Friendly Smoothies

Making diabetic-friendly smoothies is a great way to expand your horizons and think differently about how you eat. Instead of depriving yourself, you can have these healthful and delicious combinations that are easy to make and fun to enjoy. Try these diabetic smoothies and feel free to experiment with your own favorite low-carb, high energy ingredients.

1. The Great Green Smoothie

Makes 2 servings
Ingredients:
1 cup water
1/2 cup ice
1/2 cup unsweetened almond milk
1 cup raw broccoli
1 cup spinach
1 cup blueberries
2 tablespoons sunflower seeds
1 cup whole oats

Directions:
Blend the water, milk, sunflower seeds and whole oats on high until combined. Add the blueberries, broccoli and spinach and continue blending until smooth. Add the ice at the end to chill the ingredients.

Green smoothies are a staple in most healthy eating plans, and you'll find yourself craving them every once in a while.

2. Cuke and Kiwi Smoothie

Makes 2 servings
Ingredients:
1 cucumber
2 kiwis
1 cup frozen broccoli
8 ounces water
1 cup sliced peaches
1/2 cup ice

Directions:
Peel the cucumber and remove seeds. Peel the kiwi as well and add the fruit to the blender with the water. Include the sliced peaches and the ice. Blend until all the frozen items are combined and the consistency is smooth.

Remember that cucumbers are predominately water, so you'll have a looser smoothie than you expect.

3. Straw-Celery Smoothie

Makes 1 serving
Ingredients:
1 cup frozen strawberries
3 sticks of celery
1/4 cup plain yogurt
1 apple
1/2 cup water

Directions:

Peel and core the apple, ensuring seeds are removed. Chop the celery and toss into the blender with the frozen strawberries and yogurt. Cover with water and blend on high.

You may not have thought of combining strawberries and celery, but the two flavors complement each other beautifully.

4. Bloody Mary Smoothie

Makes 1 serving

Ingredients:
1 large tomato
2 stalks of celery
1 cucumber
2 tablespoons chopped red onion
1 cup plain yogurt
1/2 cup water
1 tablespoon chopped fresh cilantro
1 teaspoon Tabasco sauce

Directions:

Peel the cucumber and remove the seeds. Chop it up coarsely and combine with the tomato and celery in the blender.

Pulse those ingredients together for about 30 seconds and then add the red onion, yogurt and water.

Blend for another minute and then sprinkle with cilantro and Tabasco before drinking. Cheers.

5. Carrot and Ginger Smoothie

Makes 1 serving
Ingredients:
2 oranges, peeled
2 raw carrots, chopped
1/2 inch piece of raw ginger
1/4 cup water
1/4 cup ice

Directions:
Squeeze the juice out of the oranges and directly into the blender. Toss the fruit of the oranges in there after they have been juiced. Add the carrots and coarsely chop the ginger before adding it to the blender.

Add the water and the ice and blend until smooth. Add more water if the smoothie is too thick.

6. Thanksgiving Smoothie

Makes 2 servings
Ingredients:
1/2 cup fresh cranberries
2 fresh carrots, chopped
2 apples, peeled and cored
1 cup cooked and cooled butternut squash
1 cup water
1/4 cup chopped almonds

Directions:

This can be made as a smoothie in your blender and if you have a juicer, you can also feed the ingredients through that without the water for a thinner consistency.

In a blender, combine all the ingredients and pulse on high until everything is combined. It's a healthier version of the holiday feast.

7. Cabbage Patch Smoothie

Makes 2 servings

Ingredients:
1 cup cabbage
1 cup blueberries
1 apple
1 carrot
1 cup water
1/2 cup ice
1 tablespoon chopped fresh ginger

Directions:
Peel and core the apple, then chop it. Peel the carrot and chop that as well. Place everything inside a blender and pulse until combined and the desired level of smoothness is achieved.

Some people like to salt the cabbage before using it in a smoothie, but to keep it healthier and the fluids intact, use the leafy vegetable in its natural salt-free state.

8. Vegetable Soup Smoothie

Makes 1 serving
Ingredients:
1/2 zucchini
1/2 cucumber
1 cup broccoli florets
1 carrot
1 green apple
1 cup water
1/2 cup ice

Directions:
Peel the apple and remove the core and seeds. Combine it in the blender with the zucchini, cucumber, celery, broccoli and carrot.

After about 20 seconds, add the ice and the water and continue blending until everything is combined.

The heavy veggie flavor is sweetened considerably by the tart green apple. You'll love the fresh, healthy taste.

9. It's All Greek to Me Smoothie

Makes 2 servings
Ingredients:
1 cup cauliflower florets
2 cups cantaloupe
1 cup frozen strawberries
1 cup plain Greek yogurt
1/2 cup water

Directions:

Combine all of the ingredients and blend on high until it's as thin or frothy as you like.

The Greek yogurt will create a creamy, smooth taste that seems like a treat. The cauliflower adds a punch of fiber and works well with the fruits.

10. Veggie Madness Smoothie

Makes 2 servings

Ingredients:
1 tomato, chopped
1/3 cup chopped cucumber
2 cloves raw garlic
1 stalk celery
2 cups spinach
2 shallots, peeled
1/4 cup red bell pepper
2 cups water
1 teaspoon red pepper flakes

Directions:

This smoothie is not for the faint of heart because it packs the power of fiber and a burst of heat from the red pepper flakes. It's a who's who list of healthy vegetables, however, packed with vitamins, minerals and antioxidants.

Combine everything in a blender or food processor and pulse for three minutes until combined. The amount of nutrients and vitamins you're getting in this smoothie is bonkers, hence the name.

11. Health and Healing Smoothie

Makes 1 serving
Ingredients:
1/2 avocado
1/2 cup frozen raspberries
1/2 tablespoon coconut oil
1 cup water
1/2 teaspoon turmeric
1/2 teaspoon ginger
1 tablespoon flaxseeds

Directions:

Peel and remove the pit from the avocado. Scoop into the blender with the rest of the ingredients. Blend for about a minute until everything is combined and smooth.

The antioxidant properties in all these ingredients make this smoothie an ideal remedy for any illness. It will also build up your immune system, which is a valuable line of defense for people dealing with diabetes.

12. Eat Your Spinach Smoothie

Makes 1 serving
Ingredients:
1 apple
2 cups fresh spinach
1/2 avocado
1 cup water
1/4 cup walnuts
1/4 cup strawberries

Directions:

Peel and core the apple, making sure there are no seeds. Take the pit out of the avocado and scoop out the half that you're using.

Place everything in the blender and start blending on low for about 10 seconds. Increase the speed until everything is combined and the spinach has been shredded.

If you have a problem working spinach into your diet, this is a great solution. If you really hate it, substitute it for kale or another leafy green.

13. Kale and Cantaloupe Smoothie

Makes 2 servings
Ingredients:
2 cups kale
2 cups chopped cantaloupe
1 cup coconut water
1 tablespoon coconut flakes
1 cup ice
2 tablespoons plain yogurt

Directions:

Remove any ribs and stems from the kale and toss it in a blender with the other ingredients. Blend on high until everything is combined.

You'll love the sweet bite of the cantaloupe and how nicely it tastes with a hint of healthy coconut.

14. Pumpkin Patch Smoothie

Makes 2 servings

Ingredients:
1/2 cup unsweetened pureed pumpkin
1/2 cup raw hazelnuts
1 teaspoon cinnamon
1 teaspoon nutmeg
2 cups of spinach
2 cups coconut water

Directions:

Soak the hazelnuts for four hours before you use them in this smoothie. Pour the coconut water into the blender and add the pumpkin and spinach.

Blend together for about 30 seconds. Add the cinnamon, nutmeg and hazelnuts.

Blend for another minute or two until combined. It's like a pumpkin pie in a smoothie glass.

15. Salsa Smoothie

Makes 2 servings

Ingredients:
2 cups chopped tomatoes
1/4 cup chopped red onion
2 cloves garlic
2 lime, juiced
1 cup water
1/2 teaspoon cayenne pepper

Directions:

Juice the limes and combine all other ingredients in the blender. Pulse on high speed until blended. Use more or less cayenne depending on how spicy you want your smoothie.

Skip the tortilla chips and enjoy your salsa as a drink. This gives you all the health benefits without the corresponding dangers.

16. Pizza Smoothie

Makes 1 serving

Ingredients:
2 cups tomatoes, chopped
1/2 cup fresh basil
1 cup fresh spinach
1/4 cup chopped red pepper
2 tablespoons olive oil
1 tablespoon tamari
1 teaspoon red pepper flakes

Directions:

Combine all the ingredients in a blender and blend on medium until everything is mixed and smooth. Add a drizzle of water if the consistency is too thick.

These are some of the healthiest and most easily digested pizza toppings. Skip the pepperoni and concentrate on the veggie version instead.

17. Cucumber-Pear Smoothie

Makes 1 serving
Ingredients:
1 cucumber
2 pears
2 cups romaine lettuce
1/2 cup water
1 tablespoon flaxseed

Directions:
Peel the cucumber and scoop out the seeds. Core and peel the pears as well. Place the fruits in the blender and cover with the lettuce and the water. Add the flaxseed.

Pulse on high until everything is blended. A light, refreshing smoothie for any time of the day or night.

18. Bitter Melon Smoothie

Makes 2 servings
Ingredients:
2 bitter melons
1 kiwi
1 apple
1 tablespoon cinnamon
1 cup water
1/2 cup ice

Directions:
Peel, core and remove seeds from the bitter melons, the kiwi and the apple. Put all the ingredients in a blender and top with ice.

Pulse on high until the fruit breaks down and everything is smooth.

Bitter melon contains the substance called polypeptide-p that acts like insulin to lower blood sugar. In addition, bitter melon contains charatin, which promotes the conversion of glucose to glycogen for storage. Together, polypeptide-p and charatin can help reduce blood sugar levels effectively. Don't be intimidated by the bitter melon. Its bite is modified by the sweet kiwi and the yummy cinnamon.

19. Minty Cantaloupe Smoothie

Makes 2 servings

Ingredients:
2 cups cantaloupe
1 cup honeydew melon
1 cucumber
1 lime, juiced
1 cup fresh spinach
2 tablespoons fresh mint
1/2 cup water

Directions:
Chop the cantaloupe and melon and peel and seed the cucumber. Squeeze the lime juice into the blender and add all the ingredients. Blend on high until the ingredients are smooth and green.

The fresh taste of mint is just right when you're sipping this smoothie, which could easily be mistaken as a cocktail.

20. Nutty Blackberry Smoothie

Makes 2 servings
Ingredients:
2 cups frozen sliced peaches
1 cup blackberries
1 cup freshly squeezed orange juice
2 tablespoons fresh lemon juice
1/2 cup water
3 tablespoons coarsely chopped walnuts

Directions:
Combine everything except the walnuts in a blender. Pulse on high until combined and silky. Sprinkle the walnuts on top before you enjoy.

Look for blackberries while they are in season; they'll be plump and full and bursting with flavor.

21. Greenberry Smoothie

Makes 1 serving
Ingredients:
1/2 cup strawberries
1/2 cup blueberries
1/2 avocado
1/2 cup unsweetened almond milk
1/2 lemon, juiced
1/4 cup plain yogurt

Directions:

Peel and skin the avocado, and remove the pit. Toss into the blender with the berries, yogurt, milk and lemon juice. Blend on high until combined and smooth.

You get the best of both worlds with this smoothie; your favorite fruits as well as the healthy oil and fat from the avocado.

22. Creamsicle Smoothie

Makes 1 serving
Ingredients:
1 cup frozen peaches
1/4 cup oats
2 carrots, chopped
2 oranges, juiced
1/2 cup coconut water
1/4 cup almonds, toasted and chopped

Directions:

Roast almonds in the oven on 375 degrees for 20 minutes, then chop finely. After they have cooled, add them to your blender with all the other ingredients.

Blend on high for two or three minutes and garnish the smoothie with an orange slice.

This smoothie is like a dessert but can be enjoyed before, during and between meals.

23. Greek Grapefruit Smoothie

Makes 1 serving

Ingredients:
3 cups raw kale
1 red grapefruit, juiced
1/2 cup plain Greek yogurt
1 apple
1 cup ice

Directions:
Remove any stems or ribs from the kale and make sure the apple is cored, peeled and seeded. Place all the ingredients in the blender and combine on high for at least two or three minutes, until smooth.

You have the option of adding the grapefruit pulp to this smoothie as well, if you like a consistency that's a bit chunkier.

24. Cran-Apple Smoothie

Makes 2 servings

Ingredients:
1 gala apple
1 cup frozen cranberries
1/2 cup water
1/2 cup plain yogurt
1 teaspoon cinnamon
1 teaspoon vanilla
1/2 cup ice
1/4 cup walnuts

Directions:

Core the apple but leave the skin intact. Chop and add to the blender with cranberries, ice, water and yogurt. Blend for one minute and then add the cinnamon, vanilla and walnuts.

Blend for two more minutes until smooth. The frozen cranberries combined with the extra ice makes this smoothie seem like an ice cream treat.

25. Peachy Keen Smoothie

Makes 2 servings
Ingredients:
2 cups frozen peach slices
1 apricot
1 cup plain yogurt
1/2 cup unsweetened almond milk
1/2 cup ice
1 teaspoon grated lemon peel
1/2 lemon, juiced
1/4 cup frozen blueberries

Directions:

Remove the pit from the apricot and cut into chunks. Add it to a blender with the other ingredients. Blend on high for at least two minutes until everything is combined and the ice is broken down into a frozen concoction.

The hint of lemon in the peel is just right; not overpowering but not so subtle that you miss it.

26. Bluest of Berries Smoothie

Makes 1 serving
Ingredients:
1 cup frozen blueberries
1/2 cup frozen blackberries
1 cup unsweetened almond milk
1/4 cup whole oats

Directions:
Cover the frozen berries in a blender with the almond milk. Add the oats and blend together until combined. Add ice for a frostier consistency if preferred.

The color of this smoothie is just as appealing as the taste.

27. Nutty Pear Smoothie

Makes 1 serving
Ingredients:
2 pears
1/4 cup almonds
1 cup spinach
1/2 cup oats
1 cup unsweetened almond milk
1/2 cup ice

Directions:
Peel the pears and core them, ensuring there are no seeds or stems in the blender. Add all the other ingredients and blend together on high until everything is combined.

Allow it to rest in the refrigerator for 10 minutes before drinking.

28. Cinnamon Pear and Apple Smoothie

Makes 1 serving

Ingredients:

2 pears
1 apple
1/2 cup unsweetened almond milk
1/2 cup plain yogurt
1 teaspoon cinnamon
1/2 teaspoon nutmeg

Directions:

Core and peel the pears and apple. Chop them up roughly and place them in the blender with all the other ingredients. Combine until smooth.

Add ice to the recipe if you prefer a smoothie that's a little thicker, chunkier or colder. You can also sprinkle some cinnamon on top of the smoothie once it's finished to enjoy some extra flavor.

29. Citrus Smoothie

Makes 2 servings
Ingredients:
2 grapefruits, juiced
3 oranges, juiced
1/2 cup water
1/2 cup ice
1/2 cup fresh blueberries
1/2 cup fresh strawberries
1 sprig of mint

Directions:
Juice the citrus fruits and place the liquid in the blender. Add water, ice and fresh berries. If you elect to use frozen berries instead of fresh, you probably don't need the ice.

Blend the ingredients on high until combined. Garnish with mint.

This fresh and light smoothie will have you puckering and enjoying every bit of its sweetness.

30. Kiwi and Strawberry Smoothie

Makes 2 servings
Ingredients:
1 cup strawberries, chopped
1 kiwi, peeled and chopped
1/2 cup plain yogurt
1 cup freshly squeezed orange juice
1/2 cup ice

Directions:

Combine all the fruit and the yogurt and top with ice. Combine in the blender for about a minute.

It's sweet and good for you, and the yogurt makes it taste like a milkshake.

31. Chunky Apricot Smoothie

Makes 2 servings

Ingredients:
2 apricots
1 cup plain yogurt
1 cup freshly squeezed grapefruit juice
1 cup ice
1 tablespoon ground flaxseed

Directions:

Remove the pit from the apricots and coarsely chop before adding them to the blender. Include the other ingredients and instead of blending until smooth, do a coarse pulse, leaving some of the apricot fruit chunky.

If you prefer a smoother texture, keep blending until you get the consistency you desire.

32. Ginger and Turmeric Smoothie

Makes 1 serving

Ingredients:
1 apple
1/2 cantaloupe, chopped
1/2 teaspoon turmeric
1 teaspoon fresh ginger, grated
1/4 cup coconut milk
1/4 cup water
1 tablespoon coconut oil
2 tablespoons freshly squeezed lemon juice

Directions:
Peel, core and chop the apple before putting it into a blender. The cantaloupe should be removed from its skin. Combine all the ingredients into the blender and pulse on high until combined.

This provides a unique taste that you'll come to love.

33. Orange Juicy Smoothie

Makes 2 servings

Ingredients:
1 cup freshly squeezed orange juice
1 cup strawberries
2 peaches
2 cups ice

Directions:

Slice the peaches and remove the pits. Pour the orange juice into the blender and if you want, you can add the fruit of the orange that is leftover.

Add the peaches and the strawberries and cover the fruit with ice. Blend on high for at least one minute, until everything is combined and the consistency is smooth and frothy.

A great breakfast smoothie if you miss your regular glass of orange juice to start the day.

34. Sensational Spices Smoothie

Makes 1 serving
Ingredients:
1 pear
1 apple
1 bitter melon
1 tablespoon grated turmeric
1 tablespoon grated ginger
1 teaspoon cinnamon
2 tablespoons olive oil
1 cup water

Directions:
Wash the apple and pear, then core them and remove the seeds. Leave the skins on for the added benefit of fiber and extra nutrients.

Remove the seeds and fibers inside the bitter melon. Grate the fresh ginger and turmeric. Put some of the spices aside if you want to garnish the smoothie with them when it's ready.

Put all of the prepared ingredients into a blender and pulse on high until everything is combined. Sprinkle extra cinnamon or a bit of the ginger on top before drinking.

35. Coconut Almond Smoothie

Makes 2 servings

Ingredients:
1 cup unsweetened almond milk
1/2 cup coconut water
1 cup cubed cantaloupe pieces
1 apple
1/2 teaspoon cinnamon
1 tablespoon flaked coconut
1/2 cup ice
2 tablespoons crushed almonds

Directions:

Peel the apple and remove the core and seeds. Put the fruit in the blender with the ice and blend for about 30 seconds.

Add all the other ingredients and pulse on high speed for about a minute, until combined and smooth.

These diabetic smoothies are delicious, healthy and mindful of your sugar intake. You might think you have to sacrifice delicious things when you're managing your diabetes, but you don't. You simply have to watch you eat and get creative with how you use your favorite ingredients. Your diabetes doesn't have to limit you. Try these smoothies and get bold about trying your own combinations of fruits and vegetables in a blender.

Conclusion

Diabetic-friendly smoothies will provide you with a number of benefits. First, they'll be easy to prepare and fun to try. Second, they will be nutritious and healthy, ensuring you get the right vitamins and minerals without the added sugar. Third, they will help you keep your food cravings under control. Coupled with medication and regular exercise, eating healthy can help manage your blood sugar and in some people, it has even reversed their diabetes.

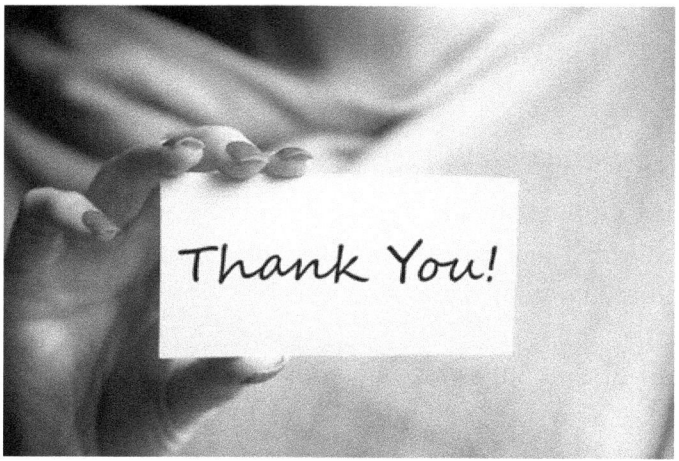

Finally, I want to thank you for reading my book. If you enjoyed the book, please share your thoughts and post a review on the book retailer's website. It would be greatly appreciated!

Best wishes,
Amanda Hopkins

Check Out My Other Books

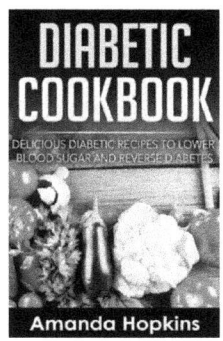

Diabetic Cookbook: Delicious Diabetic Recipes to Lower Blood Sugar and Reverse Diabetes

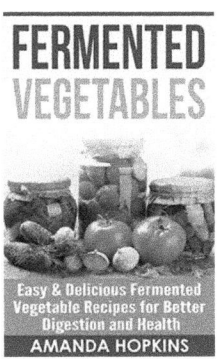

Fermented Vegetables: Easy & Delicious Fermented Vegetable Recipes for Better Digestion and Health

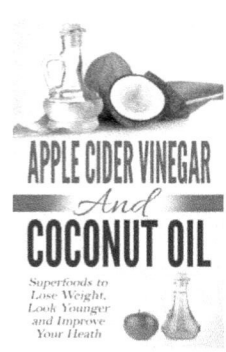

Apple Cider Vinegar and Coconut Oil: Superfoods to Lose Weight, Look Younger and Improve Your Heath

Lightning Source UK Ltd.
Milton Keynes UK
UKHW020031060721
386683UK00002B/161